Blood Pres

Record your readings in this
on your next visit so that he sne can easily diagnose your
condition and monitor your progress.

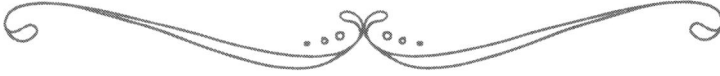

Name:.. DOB:...

Doctor's Name:.. ☎ ....

Why maintaining a blood pressure log is important:

- To see for yourself how your treatment is working for you
  - are lifestyle changes or medication having any effect on your blood pressure

- It can help with early diagnosis of high blood pressure

- To alert you/your doctor to unexpected changes in your readings,
  helping them to make changes to or adjust your medication

- To help identify white coat hypertension
  - where the pressure is markedly higher due to anxiety about seeing a doctor

---

What do the numbers mean?

- Blood pressure is classified into two different categories which are systolic and diastolic

- The *systolic* blood pressure refers to the pressure in your blood vessels when your *heart beats*

- The *diastolic* blood pressure refers to the pressure in your blood vessels when your *heart rests* between beats

Blood Pressure Categories

BLOOD PRESSURE CATEGORY	SYSTOLIC mm Hg (upper number)		DIASTOLIC mm Hg (lower number)
NORMAL	LESS THAN 120	and	LESS THAN 80
ELEVATED	120 - 129	and	LESS THAN 80
HIGH BLOOD PRESSURE (HYPERTENSION) STAGE 1	130 - 139	or	80 - 89
HIGH BLOOD PRESSURE (HYPERTENSION) STAGE 2	140 OR HIGHER	or	90 OR HIGHER
HYPERTENSION CRISIS (Consult your doctor immediately!)	HIGHER THAN 180	and /or	HIGHER THAN 120

Helpful notes:

(BP = Blood Pressure)

1. *Never check your BP first thing in the morning.*
   Why? Because an increase of BP is part of the waking up system.

2. Similarly, a decrease in BP is part of the "falling asleep" system, so to get a baseline, the ***best time to take your BP is before going to sleep.***

3. ***Don't take your BP*** if you are angry, happy, or pushing a fridge.
   To pump blood through clenched muscles, your BP needs to go up, so it is not meaningful if your muscles are clenched in anger, in mirth or in effort.

4. If your BP is high when you are completely relaxed, then ***you really have a problem.***

5. ***Things that increase your BP:*** fat (weight), caffeine, nicotine, salt and excess alcohol.

6. ***Things that reduce your BP:*** genetics, low salt, exercise and weight loss.

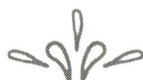

DATE	TIME		SYSTOLIC BP (upper number)	PULSE (beats per minute)	NOTES (e.g. medication changes, feeling unwell, activities)
	am	pm	DIASTOLIC BP (lower number)		
example: 07/03 2019	9:15		127	85	Feeling good, started taking new medication
	(am)	pm	84		
					....
	am	pm			
					....
	am	pm			
					....
	am	pm			
					....
	am	pm			
					....
	am	pm			
					....
	am	pm			
					....
	am	pm			
					....
	am	pm			
Average Systolic				Average bpm	
Average Diastolic					

DATE	TIME		SYSTOLIC BP (upper number) DIASTOLIC BP (lower number)	PULSE (beats per minute)	NOTES (e.g. medication changes, feeling unwell, activities)
	am	pm			....
	am	pm			....
	am	pm			....
	am	pm			....
	am	pm			....
	am	pm			....
	am	pm			....
	am	pm			....
	am	pm			....
Average Systolic				Average bpm	
Average Diastolic					

DATE	TIME		SYSTOLIC BP (upper number)	PULSE (beats per minute)	NOTES (e.g. medication changes, feeling unwell, activities)
	am	pm	DIASTOLIC BP (lower number)		
					....
	am	pm			
					....
	am	pm			
					....
	am	pm			
					....
	am	pm			
					....
	am	pm			
					....
	am	pm			
					....
	am	pm			
					....
	am	pm			
					....
	am	pm			
Average Systolic				Average bpm	
Average Diastolic					

DATE	TIME		SYSTOLIC BP (upper number)	PULSE (beats per minute)	NOTES (e.g. medication changes, feeling unwell, activities)
	am	pm	DIASTOLIC BP (lower number)		
					....
	am	pm			....
					....
	am	pm			....
					....
	am	pm			....
					....
	am	pm			....
					....
	am	pm			....
					....
	am	pm			....
					....
	am	pm			....
					....
	am	pm			....
					....
	am	pm			....
Average Systolic				Average bpm	
Average Diastolic					

DATE	TIME		SYSTOLIC BP (upper number) DIASTOLIC BP (lower number)	PULSE (beats per minute)	NOTES (e.g. medication changes, feeling unwell, activities)
	am	pm			....
	am	pm			....
	am	pm			....
	am	pm			....
	am	pm			....
	am	pm			....
	am	pm			....
	am	pm			....
	am	pm			....
Average Systolic				Average bpm	
Average Diastolic					

DATE	TIME		SYSTOLIC BP (upper number) DIASTOLIC BP (lower number)	PULSE (beats per minute)	NOTES (e.g. medication changes, feeling unwell, activities)
	am	pm			....
	am	pm			....
	am	pm			....
	am	pm			....
	am	pm			....
	am	pm			....
	am	pm			....
	am	pm			....
	am	pm			....
Average Systolic				Average bpm	
Average Diastolic					

DATE	TIME		SYSTOLIC BP (upper number)	PULSE (beats per minute)	NOTES (e.g. medication changes, feeling unwell, activities)
	am	pm	DIASTOLIC BP (lower number)		
					....
	am	pm			....
					....
	am	pm			....
					....
	am	pm			....
					....
	am	pm			....
					....
	am	pm			....
					....
	am	pm			....
					....
	am	pm			....
					....
	am	pm			....
					....
	am	pm			....
Average Systolic				Average bpm	
Average Diastolic					

DATE	TIME		SYSTOLIC BP (upper number) DIASTOLIC BP (lower number)	PULSE (beats per minute)	NOTES (e.g. medication changes, feeling unwell, activities)
	am	pm			....
	am	pm			....
	am	pm			....
	am	pm			....
	am	pm			....
	am	pm			....
	am	pm			....
	am	pm			....
	am	pm			....
Average Systolic				Average bpm	
Average Diastolic					

DATE	TIME		SYSTOLIC BP (upper number) DIASTOLIC BP (lower number)	PULSE (beats per minute)	NOTES (e.g. medication changes, feeling unwell, activities)
	am	pm			....
	am	pm			....
	am	pm			....
	am	pm			....
	am	pm			....
	am	pm			....
	am	pm			....
	am	pm			....
	am	pm			....
Average Systolic				Average bpm	
Average Diastolic					

DATE	TIME		SYSTOLIC BP (upper number)	PULSE (beats per minute)	NOTES (e.g. medication changes, feeling unwell, activities)
	am	pm	DIASTOLIC BP (lower number)		
					....
	am	pm			....
					....
	am	pm			....
					....
	am	pm			....
					....
	am	pm			....
					....
	am	pm			....
					....
	am	pm			....
					....
	am	pm			....
					....
	am	pm			....
					....
	am	pm			....
Average Systolic				Average bpm	
Average Diastolic					

DATE	TIME		SYSTOLIC BP (upper number)	PULSE (beats per minute)	NOTES (e.g. medication changes, feeling unwell, activities)
	am	pm	DIASTOLIC BP (lower number)		
	am	pm			....
	am	pm			....
	am	pm			....
	am	pm			....
	am	pm			....
	am	pm			....
	am	pm			....
	am	pm			....
	am	pm			....
Average Systolic				Average bpm	
Average Diastolic					

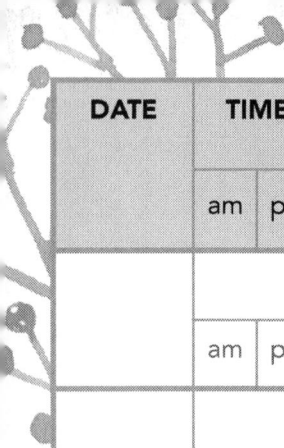

DATE	TIME		SYSTOLIC BP (upper number)	PULSE (beats per minute)	NOTES (e.g. medication changes, feeling unwell, activities)
	am	pm	DIASTOLIC BP (lower number)		
					....
	am	pm			....
					....
	am	pm			....
					....
	am	pm			....
					....
	am	pm			....
					....
	am	pm			....
					....
	am	pm			....
					....
	am	pm			....
					....
	am	pm			....
					....
	am	pm			....
Average Systolic				Average bpm	
Average Diastolic					

DATE	TIME		SYSTOLIC BP (upper number)	PULSE (beats per minute)	NOTES (e.g. medication changes, feeling unwell, activities)
	am	pm	DIASTOLIC BP (lower number)		
					....
	am	pm			....
					....
	am	pm			....
					....
	am	pm			....
					....
	am	pm			....
					....
	am	pm			....
					....
	am	pm			....
					....
	am	pm			....
					....
	am	pm			....
					....
	am	pm			....
Average Systolic				Average bpm	
Average Diastolic					

DATE	TIME		SYSTOLIC BP (upper number) DIASTOLIC BP (lower number)	PULSE (beats per minute)	NOTES (e.g. medication changes, feeling unwell, activities)
	am	pm			....
	am	pm			....
	am	pm			....
	am	pm			....
	am	pm			....
	am	pm			....
	am	pm			....
	am	pm			....
	am	pm			....
Average Systolic				Average bpm	
Average Diastolic					

DATE	TIME		SYSTOLIC BP (upper number)	PULSE (beats per minute)	NOTES (e.g. medication changes, feeling unwell, activities)
	am	pm	DIASTOLIC BP (lower number)		
	am	pm			....
	am	pm			....
	am	pm			....
	am	pm			....
	am	pm			....
	am	pm			....
	am	pm			....
	am	pm			....
	am	pm			....
Average Systolic				Average bpm	
Average Diastolic					

DATE	TIME		SYSTOLIC BP (upper number) DIASTOLIC BP (lower number)	PULSE (beats per minute)	NOTES (e.g. medication changes, feeling unwell, activities)
	am	pm			....
	am	pm			....
	am	pm			....
	am	pm			....
	am	pm			....
	am	pm			....
	am	pm			....
	am	pm			....
	am	pm			....
Average Systolic				Average bpm	
Average Diastolic					

DATE	TIME		SYSTOLIC BP (upper number)	PULSE (beats per minute)	NOTES (e.g. medication changes, feeling unwell, activities)
	am	pm	DIASTOLIC BP (lower number)		
	am	pm			....
	am	pm			....
	am	pm			....
	am	pm			....
	am	pm			....
	am	pm			....
	am	pm			....
	am	pm			....
	am	pm			....
Average Systolic				Average bpm	
Average Diastolic					

DATE	TIME		SYSTOLIC BP (upper number)	PULSE (beats per minute)	NOTES (e.g. medication changes, feeling unwell, activities)
	am	pm	DIASTOLIC BP (lower number)		
	am	pm			....
	am	pm			....
	am	pm			....
	am	pm			....
	am	pm			....
	am	pm			....
	am	pm			....
	am	pm			....
	am	pm			....
Average Systolic				Average bpm	
Average Diastolic					

DATE	TIME		SYSTOLIC BP (upper number) DIASTOLIC BP (lower number)	PULSE (beats per minute)	NOTES (e.g. medication changes, feeling unwell, activities)
	am	pm			....
	am	pm			....
	am	pm			....
	am	pm			....
	am	pm			....
	am	pm			....
	am	pm			....
	am	pm			....
	am	pm			....
Average Systolic				Average bpm	
Average Diastolic					

DATE	TIME		SYSTOLIC BP (upper number) DIASTOLIC BP (lower number)	PULSE (beats per minute)	NOTES (e.g. medication changes, feeling unwell, activities)
	am	pm			....
	am	pm			....
	am	pm			....
	am	pm			....
	am	pm			....
	am	pm			....
	am	pm			....
	am	pm			....
	am	pm			....
Average Systolic				Average bpm	
Average Diastolic					

DATE	TIME		SYSTOLIC BP (upper number)	PULSE (beats per minute)	NOTES (e.g. medication changes, feeling unwell, activities)
	am	pm	DIASTOLIC BP (lower number)		
	am	pm			....
	am	pm			....
	am	pm			....
	am	pm			....
	am	pm			....
	am	pm			....
	am	pm			....
	am	pm			....
	am	pm			....
Average Systolic				Average bpm	
Average Diastolic					

DATE	TIME		SYSTOLIC BP (upper number)	PULSE (beats per minute)	NOTES (e.g. medication changes, feeling unwell, activities)
	am	pm	DIASTOLIC BP (lower number)		
					....
	am	pm			....
					....
	am	pm			....
					....
	am	pm			....
					....
	am	pm			....
					....
	am	pm			....
					....
	am	pm			....
					....
	am	pm			....
					....
	am	pm			....
					....
	am	pm			....
Average Systolic				Average bpm	
Average Diastolic					

DATE	TIME		SYSTOLIC BP (upper number)	PULSE (beats per minute)	NOTES (e.g. medication changes, feeling unwell, activities)
	am	pm	DIASTOLIC BP (lower number)		
					....
	am	pm			....
					....
	am	pm			....
					....
	am	pm			....
					....
	am	pm			....
					....
	am	pm			....
					....
	am	pm			....
					....
	am	pm			....
					....
	am	pm			....
					....
	am	pm			....
Average Systolic				Average bpm	
Average Diastolic					

DATE	TIME		SYSTOLIC BP (upper number)	PULSE (beats per minute)	NOTES (e.g. medication changes, feeling unwell, activities)
	am	pm	DIASTOLIC BP (lower number)		
	am	pm			....
	am	pm			....
	am	pm			....
	am	pm			....
	am	pm			....
	am	pm			....
	am	pm			....
	am	pm			....
	am	pm			....
Average Systolic				Average bpm	
Average Diastolic					

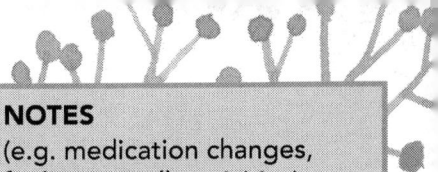

DATE	TIME		SYSTOLIC BP (upper number)	PULSE (beats per minute)	NOTES (e.g. medication changes, feeling unwell, activities)
	am	pm	DIASTOLIC BP (lower number)		
	am	pm			....
	am	pm			....
	am	pm			....
	am	pm			....
	am	pm			....
	am	pm			....
	am	pm			....
	am	pm			....
	am	pm			....
Average Systolic				Average bpm	
Average Diastolic					

DATE	TIME		SYSTOLIC BP (upper number)	PULSE (beats per minute)	NOTES (e.g. medication changes, feeling unwell, activities)
	am	pm	DIASTOLIC BP (lower number)		
	am	pm			....
	am	pm			....
	am	pm			....
	am	pm			....
	am	pm			....
	am	pm			....
	am	pm			....
	am	pm			....
	am	pm			....
Average Systolic				Average bpm	
Average Diastolic					

DATE	TIME		SYSTOLIC BP (upper number) DIASTOLIC BP (lower number)	PULSE (beats per minute)	NOTES (e.g. medication changes, feeling unwell, activities)
	am	pm			....
	am	pm			....
	am	pm			....
	am	pm			....
	am	pm			....
	am	pm			....
	am	pm			....
	am	pm			....
	am	pm			....
Average Systolic				Average bpm	
Average Diastolic					

DATE	TIME		SYSTOLIC BP (upper number) DIASTOLIC BP (lower number)	PULSE (beats per minute)	NOTES (e.g. medication changes, feeling unwell, activities)
	am	pm			....
	am	pm			....
	am	pm			....
	am	pm			....
	am	pm			....
	am	pm			....
	am	pm			....
	am	pm			....
	am	pm			....
Average Systolic				Average bpm	
Average Diastolic					

DATE	TIME		SYSTOLIC BP (upper number)	PULSE (beats per minute)	NOTES (e.g. medication changes, feeling unwell, activities)
	am	pm	DIASTOLIC BP (lower number)		
					....
	am	pm			
					....
	am	pm			
					....
	am	pm			
					....
	am	pm			
					....
	am	pm			
					....
	am	pm			
					....
	am	pm			
					....
	am	pm			
					....
	am	pm			
Average Systolic				Average bpm	
Average Diastolic					

DATE	TIME		SYSTOLIC BP (upper number)	PULSE (beats per minute)	NOTES (e.g. medication changes, feeling unwell, activities)
	am	pm	DIASTOLIC BP (lower number)		
	am	pm			....
	am	pm			....
	am	pm			....
	am	pm			....
	am	pm			....
	am	pm			....
	am	pm			....
	am	pm			....
	am	pm			....
Average Systolic				Average bpm	
Average Diastolic					

DATE	TIME		SYSTOLIC BP (upper number) / DIASTOLIC BP (lower number)	PULSE (beats per minute)	NOTES (e.g. medication changes, feeling unwell, activities)
	am	pm			....
	am	pm			....
	am	pm			....
	am	pm			....
	am	pm			....
	am	pm			....
	am	pm			....
	am	pm			....
	am	pm			....
Average Systolic				Average bpm	
Average Diastolic					

DATE	TIME		SYSTOLIC BP (upper number) DIASTOLIC BP (lower number)	PULSE (beats per minute)	NOTES (e.g. medication changes, feeling unwell, activities)
	am	pm			....
	am	pm			....
	am	pm			....
	am	pm			....
	am	pm			....
	am	pm			....
	am	pm			....
	am	pm			....
	am	pm			....
Average Systolic				Average bpm	
Average Diastolic					

DATE	TIME		SYSTOLIC BP (upper number) / DIASTOLIC BP (lower number)	PULSE (beats per minute)	NOTES (e.g. medication changes, feeling unwell, activities)
	am	pm			....
	am	pm			....
	am	pm			....
	am	pm			....
	am	pm			....
	am	pm			....
	am	pm			....
	am	pm			....
	am	pm			....
Average Systolic				Average bpm	
Average Diastolic					

DATE	TIME		SYSTOLIC BP (upper number) DIASTOLIC BP (lower number)	PULSE (beats per minute)	NOTES (e.g. medication changes, feeling unwell, activities)
	am	pm			....
	am	pm			....
	am	pm			....
	am	pm			....
	am	pm			....
	am	pm			....
	am	pm			....
	am	pm			....
	am	pm			....
Average Systolic				Average bpm	
Average Diastolic					

DATE	TIME		SYSTOLIC BP (upper number) / DIASTOLIC BP (lower number)	PULSE (beats per minute)	NOTES (e.g. medication changes, feeling unwell, activities)
	am	pm			....
	am	pm			....
	am	pm			....
	am	pm			....
	am	pm			....
	am	pm			....
	am	pm			....
	am	pm			....
	am	pm			....
Average Systolic				Average bpm	
Average Diastolic					

DATE	TIME		SYSTOLIC BP (upper number) DIASTOLIC BP (lower number)	PULSE (beats per minute)	NOTES (e.g. medication changes, feeling unwell, activities)
	am	pm			....
	am	pm			....
	am	pm			....
	am	pm			....
	am	pm			....
	am	pm			....
	am	pm			....
	am	pm			....
	am	pm			....
Average Systolic				Average bpm	
Average Diastolic					

DATE	TIME		SYSTOLIC BP (upper number)	PULSE (beats per minute)	NOTES (e.g. medication changes, feeling unwell, activities)
	am	pm	DIASTOLIC BP (lower number)		
					....
	am	pm			....
					....
	am	pm			....
					....
	am	pm			....
					....
	am	pm			....
					....
	am	pm			....
					....
	am	pm			....
					....
	am	pm			....
					....
	am	pm			....
					....
	am	pm			....
Average Systolic				Average bpm	
Average Diastolic					

DATE	TIME		SYSTOLIC BP (upper number) DIASTOLIC BP (lower number)	PULSE (beats per minute)	NOTES (e.g. medication changes, feeling unwell, activities)
	am	pm			....
	am	pm			....
	am	pm			....
	am	pm			....
	am	pm			....
	am	pm			....
	am	pm			....
	am	pm			....
	am	pm			....
Average Systolic				Average bpm	
Average Diastolic					

DATE	TIME		SYSTOLIC BP (upper number)	PULSE (beats per minute)	NOTES (e.g. medication changes, feeling unwell, activities)
	am	pm	DIASTOLIC BP (lower number)		
					....
	am	pm			
					....
	am	pm			
					....
	am	pm			
					....
	am	pm			
					....
	am	pm			
					....
	am	pm			
					....
	am	pm			
					....
	am	pm			
					....
	am	pm			
Average Systolic				Average bpm	
Average Diastolic					

DATE	TIME		SYSTOLIC BP (upper number)	PULSE (beats per minute)	NOTES (e.g. medication changes, feeling unwell, activities)
	am	pm	**DIASTOLIC BP** (lower number)		
					....
	am	pm			....
					....
	am	pm			....
					....
	am	pm			....
					....
	am	pm			....
					....
	am	pm			....
					....
	am	pm			....
					....
	am	pm			....
					....
	am	pm			....
					....
	am	pm			....
Average Systolic				Average bpm	
Average Diastolic					

DATE	TIME		SYSTOLIC BP (upper number)	PULSE (beats per minute)	NOTES (e.g. medication changes, feeling unwell, activities)
	am	pm	DIASTOLIC BP (lower number)		
					....
	am	pm			
					....
	am	pm			
					....
	am	pm			
					....
	am	pm			
					....
	am	pm			
					....
	am	pm			
					....
	am	pm			
					....
	am	pm			
					....
	am	pm			
Average Systolic				Average bpm	
Average Diastolic					

DATE	TIME		SYSTOLIC BP (upper number)	PULSE (beats per minute)	NOTES (e.g. medication changes, feeling unwell, activities)
	am	pm	DIASTOLIC BP (lower number)		
					....
	am	pm			
					....
	am	pm			
					....
	am	pm			
					....
	am	pm			
					....
	am	pm			
					....
	am	pm			
					....
	am	pm			
					....
	am	pm			
					....
	am	pm			
Average Systolic				Average bpm	
Average Diastolic					

DATE	TIME		SYSTOLIC BP (upper number) DIASTOLIC BP (lower number)	PULSE (beats per minute)	NOTES (e.g. medication changes, feeling unwell, activities)
	am	pm			....
	am	pm			....
	am	pm			....
	am	pm			....
	am	pm			....
	am	pm			....
	am	pm			....
	am	pm			....
	am	pm			....
Average Systolic				Average bpm	
Average Diastolic					

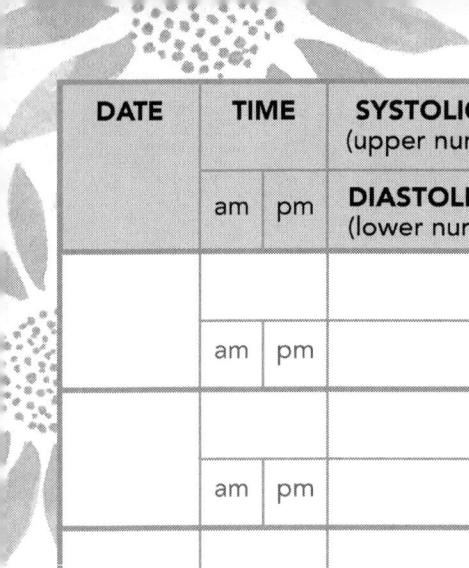

DATE	TIME		SYSTOLIC BP (upper number) DIASTOLIC BP (lower number)	PULSE (beats per minute)	NOTES (e.g. medication changes, feeling unwell, activities)
	am	pm			
	am	pm			....
	am	pm			....
	am	pm			....
	am	pm			....
	am	pm			....
	am	pm			....
	am	pm			....
	am	pm			....
	am	pm			....
Average Systolic				Average bpm	
Average Diastolic					

DATE	TIME		SYSTOLIC BP (upper number) DIASTOLIC BP (lower number)	PULSE (beats per minute)	NOTES (e.g. medication changes, feeling unwell, activities)
	am	pm			....
	am	pm			....
	am	pm			....
	am	pm			....
	am	pm			....
	am	pm			....
	am	pm			....
	am	pm			....
	am	pm			....
Average Systolic				Average bpm	
Average Diastolic					

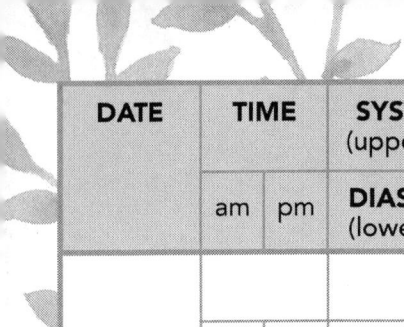

DATE	TIME		SYSTOLIC BP (upper number) DIASTOLIC BP (lower number)	PULSE (beats per minute)	NOTES (e.g. medication changes, feeling unwell, activities)
	am	pm			....
	am	pm			....
	am	pm			....
	am	pm			....
	am	pm			....
	am	pm			....
	am	pm			....
	am	pm			....
	am	pm			....
Average Systolic				Average bpm	
Average Diastolic					

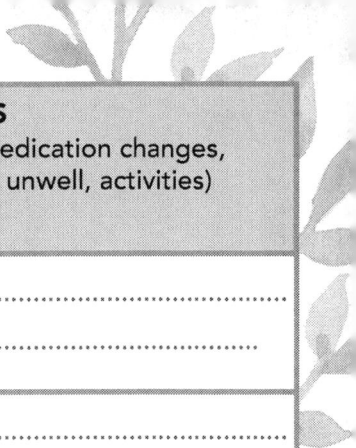

DATE	TIME		SYSTOLIC BP (upper number) DIASTOLIC BP (lower number)	PULSE (beats per minute)	NOTES (e.g. medication changes, feeling unwell, activities)
	am	pm			....
	am	pm			....
	am	pm			....
	am	pm			....
	am	pm			....
	am	pm			....
	am	pm			....
	am	pm			....
	am	pm			....
Average Systolic				Average bpm	
Average Diastolic					

DATE	TIME		SYSTOLIC BP (upper number) DIASTOLIC BP (lower number)	PULSE (beats per minute)	NOTES (e.g. medication changes, feeling unwell, activities)
	am	pm			....
	am	pm			....
	am	pm			....
	am	pm			....
	am	pm			....
	am	pm			....
	am	pm			....
	am	pm			....
	am	pm			....
Average Systolic				Average bpm	
Average Diastolic					

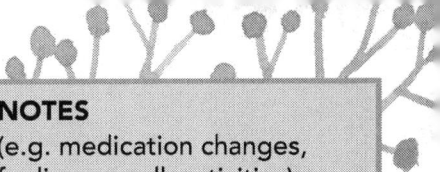

DATE	TIME		SYSTOLIC BP (upper number) DIASTOLIC BP (lower number)	PULSE (beats per minute)	NOTES (e.g. medication changes, feeling unwell, activities)
	am	pm			....
	am	pm			....
	am	pm			....
	am	pm			....
	am	pm			....
	am	pm			....
	am	pm			....
	am	pm			....
	am	pm			....
Average Systolic				Average bpm	
Average Diastolic					

DATE	TIME		SYSTOLIC BP (upper number)	PULSE (beats per minute)	NOTES (e.g. medication changes, feeling unwell, activities)
	am	pm	DIASTOLIC BP (lower number)		
	am	pm			....
	am	pm			....
	am	pm			....
	am	pm			....
	am	pm			....
	am	pm			....
	am	pm			....
	am	pm			....
	am	pm			....
Average Systolic				Average bpm	
Average Diastolic					

DATE	TIME		SYSTOLIC BP (upper number)	PULSE (beats per minute)	NOTES (e.g. medication changes, feeling unwell, activities)
	am	pm	DIASTOLIC BP (lower number)		
					....
	am	pm			....
					....
	am	pm			....
					....
	am	pm			....
					....
	am	pm			....
					....
	am	pm			....
					....
	am	pm			....
					....
	am	pm			....
					....
	am	pm			....
					....
	am	pm			....
Average Systolic				Average bpm	
Average Diastolic					

DATE	TIME		SYSTOLIC BP (upper number) DIASTOLIC BP (lower number)	PULSE (beats per minute)	NOTES (e.g. medication changes, feeling unwell, activities)
	am	pm			
					....
	am	pm			....
					....
	am	pm			....
					....
	am	pm			....
					....
	am	pm			....
					....
	am	pm			....
					....
	am	pm			....
					....
	am	pm			....
					....
	am	pm			....
					....
	am	pm			....
Average Systolic				Average bpm	
Average Diastolic					

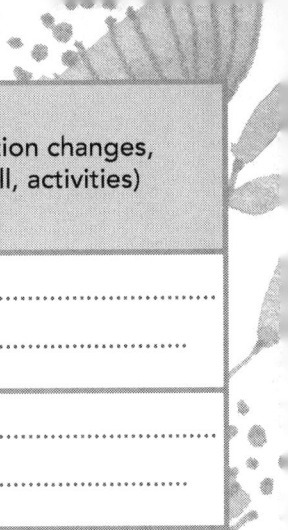

DATE	TIME		SYSTOLIC BP (upper number)	PULSE (beats per minute)	NOTES (e.g. medication changes, feeling unwell, activities)
	am	pm	DIASTOLIC BP (lower number)		
					....
	am	pm			....
					....
	am	pm			....
					....
	am	pm			....
					....
	am	pm			....
					....
	am	pm			....
					....
	am	pm			....
					....
	am	pm			....
					....
	am	pm			....
					....
	am	pm			....
Average Systolic				Average bpm	
Average Diastolic					

DATE	TIME		SYSTOLIC BP (upper number) / DIASTOLIC BP (lower number)	PULSE (beats per minute)	NOTES (e.g. medication changes, feeling unwell, activities)
	am	pm			....
	am	pm			....
	am	pm			....
	am	pm			....
	am	pm			....
	am	pm			....
	am	pm			....
	am	pm			....
	am	pm			....
Average Systolic				Average bpm	
Average Diastolic					

DATE	TIME		SYSTOLIC BP (upper number)	PULSE (beats per minute)	NOTES (e.g. medication changes, feeling unwell, activities)
	am	pm	DIASTOLIC BP (lower number)		
					....
	am	pm			....
					....
	am	pm			....
					....
	am	pm			....
					....
	am	pm			....
					....
	am	pm			....
					....
	am	pm			....
					....
	am	pm			....
					....
	am	pm			....
					....
	am	pm			....
Average Systolic				Average bpm	
Average Diastolic					

DATE	TIME		SYSTOLIC BP (upper number) DIASTOLIC BP (lower number)	PULSE (beats per minute)	NOTES (e.g. medication changes, feeling unwell, activities)
	am	pm			
	am	pm			....
	am	pm			....
	am	pm			....
	am	pm			....
	am	pm			....
	am	pm			....
	am	pm			....
	am	pm			....
Average Systolic				Average bpm	
Average Diastolic					

DATE	TIME		SYSTOLIC BP (upper number)	PULSE (beats per minute)	NOTES (e.g. medication changes, feeling unwell, activities)
	am	pm	DIASTOLIC BP (lower number)		
					....
	am	pm			....
					....
	am	pm			....
					....
	am	pm			....
					....
	am	pm			....
					....
	am	pm			....
					....
	am	pm			....
					....
	am	pm			....
					....
	am	pm			....
					....
	am	pm			....
Average Systolic				Average bpm	
Average Diastolic					

DATE	TIME		SYSTOLIC BP (upper number)	PULSE (beats per minute)	NOTES (e.g. medication changes, feeling unwell, activities)
	am	pm	DIASTOLIC BP (lower number)		
					....
	am	pm			
					....
	am	pm			
					....
	am	pm			
					....
	am	pm			
					....
	am	pm			
					....
	am	pm			
					....
	am	pm			
					....
	am	pm			
					....
	am	pm			
Average Systolic				Average bpm	
Average Diastolic					

Made in the USA
Las Vegas, NV
12 December 2022